More Praise for *Slow Now with Clear ~~Skies~~*

I must/ slow down, touch earth, find/ the smooth stone in my pocket...
These lines are at the heart of both Julene Tripp Weaver's poem,
"Safe Space," and her necessary poetry collection. Weaver uses
images from her own life and the viruses that plague our world
to witness suffering. And to acknowledge that all of us have been
changed over the Covid years. *Everyone lives on a spectrum/ of
health and neuroticism*, she tells us.

She offers no easy answers to how we might heal in a dangerous
world when even our closest relationships might betray us.
My mother never enters at the right/ time, even in my dreams, she
confides. Yet she writes that all of us can find *back doors/ into the
body* after illness, loss and the hauntings of memory.

In post-pandemic America, this is the book I needed to read.
Weaver, an herbalist, knows we and the earth can heal together.
Find channels that soothe. ...Send anxiety into the earth. One of these
channels is poetry.

The title of the collection comes from the final line of the poem
"I've Lived Through One War." She rallies us with the lines: *We
must ask/ new questions, find unconventional answers...It's time/for
massive change.../ Our planet, slow now with clear skies.*

—Joanne M. Clarkson, author of *Hospice House*

Slow
Now
with
Clear
Skies

Slow
Now
with
Clear
Skies

JULENE
TRIPP
WEAVER

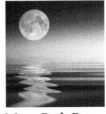

MoonPath Press

Poetry
ISBN 978-1-936657-84-1

Cover art: *what we make it* (detail), © 2021 By Clare Johnson
Watercolor on fine art print of dip pen & India ink drawing, 8.5 x 4.75 inches. From series originally made for public art, commissioned by City of Seattle Office of Arts & Culture. To see more of Clare's work, please visit www.clarejohnson.com

Author photo: Laurie Smith

Book design: Tonya Namura, using Corporate A Condensed

Library of Congress Cataloging-in-Publication Data
Author: Weaver, Julene Tripp
Title: *Slow Now with Clear Skies*
LCCN: 2024903304
Subject: Poetry

.

MoonPath Press, an imprint of Concrete Wolf Poetry Series, is dedicated to publishing the finest poets living in the U.S. Pacific Northwest.

MoonPath Press
c/o Concrete Wolf
PO Box 2220
Newport, OR 97365-0163

MoonPathPress@gmail.com
http://MoonPathPress.com

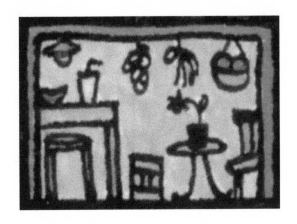

For my pandemic pal partner who helps me thrive.

For my family. My mother. My father.

For my beloved sister, who gives so much, including the continuation of our family.

For my great grandmother, and all the ancestors, who gave us life despite the toll.

For everyone who experienced loss during COVID.

Contents

Slow
Now
with
Clear
Skies

I: Fire Burns
Our Tomorrows

In a time of destruction, create something.
A poem. A parade. A community. A vow.
A moral principle. One Peaceful moment.

–Maxine Hong Kingston,
The Fifth Book of Peace

Bus Stop in San Antonio: AWP Off Site

He says I've been sent to test him,
that he's a good person so he will pass the test.
That's good.   The word schizophrenia
            lands in my brain.

He says I will act like I don't know
            what he's talking about, it's a test
of his character   tells me
            he won't hurt me.

People like you have cars.
He's black. I'm white. He's right.
I'm traveling, so I don't have a car.
He asks if I have a car at home. *I do.*

He asks why I'm taking the bus,
            reminds me, he won't hurt me.
I explain, *I lived in New York, the city,*
I'm used to public buses.

I don't fit the expectation for a white
woman with white hair, a tourist at a conference,
to wait at a bus stop in any sprawling city.
            I'm not feeble, I say.

He asks what that means.
I don't need a walker, I motion to my feet,
            sturdy. But are they? I get leg cramps.
Don't you have that—he puts his hand to his mouth

his other hand motions pushing buttons, *Uber,* he says, or...
I pull out my phone, *Lyft?* Then explain,
            I don't get data without Wi-Fi
so I take the bus or walk. Because I get texts

we look up the schedule, it's 8:48, the bus
        is due at 9:21. Agitated, he's already
waited a half-hour, says he's been up
since dawn, at a construction job.

Heading to his sister's place for the night.
        Homeless. *I'm glad you have a place to stay.*
We board the bus, sit a seat apart,
he makes sure I get off at the right stop.

We wave goodbye, I exit for the vegan café,
        healthy food and a poetry reading.
He travels on, safe for tonight.
        Missing the last bus, I walk back to the hotel.

People like me aren't expected
        to ride a bus. To walk the lonely
streets. To meet those who provide the labor
        that builds our cities.

Fires Burn Our Tomorrows

I'm grateful for that final box
of nectarines from Rama Farm
late summer, before the fire
burned their buildings to the ground,
swept through their orchard.

The inner heat, those oh-so-sweet
nectarines warmed me though
a blistering year, we know
all has changed—we will ourselves
into this new world, climate in disarray

a world filled with disbelievers—a wild
and free world where only the grounding
of cherries, peaches, nectarines, melons,
the countdown of fruits from early wild
salmonberries, raspberries, blackberries,

then blueberries, will buoy us. Fields
swelter taking our bounty, our tears
alive with sorrow—only the sweet
fruit of summer will save us—captured
savor against winter's cold ice.

We are an ungrateful tide, expressing
disbelief against this earth's plenum—
bountiful as a basket of luscious ripe
strawberries—a variety that no longer
exists—so many children will burn

in our fires of disbelief. They will never
know that first taste, the burst and pop
that makes us smile—what we
remember that protects us from storms
that steal tomorrows pleasure.

Food Chain

When it is time to die—
as if we can count the time to the inevitable
barred from the knowledge of the stars—
the moon and planets shift into alignment
with secret knowledge.

All life cracked in the cell waiting
for moisture to release what is stone hard.
We swallow pits—death grows its own path
of resilience—how much can we absorb
of immeasurable sustenance.

Circumstances of nations prevail—
the economics of soy or corn
overrides the necessity of potatoes.
Empty lots, the push of law
decides what seeds survive,

will be cloned or radiated, what nuclear
genocide we ingest day-in day-out.
We must fight back, preserve the wild,
allow insects to live their natural lives
harmonious nature to swallow us into her fold.

Daily Caution During a Pandemic

Do we go to the store for pasta,
the one and only item we need,
or not? What is the chance
of catching COVID-19?

How many in my local market
are carriers, am I protecting them,
or me? Aware of every sniffle,
sneeze, cough, the breath of my

lover in my face when we go to
bed, I turn away, push my back
up against him. He is my pandemic
pal, lucky to have a body connection,

not alone. We work from home,
get along, this is not our first test,
not even the second in our long
history. May we continue to thrive.

Pupal Soup

In a dark time, the eye begins to see.
                    —Theodore Roethke

Oh Theodore, had you been here
with us these past years—
to sit inside your greenhouse—so many
sad, a dark time said to be surreal—a lie,
but yes, out of the ordinary, nature
has always had its way with us—
eruptions, floods, fire—the cycle comes
round with our raw commercialization,
too many choices. We take without care—
blow off mountain tops, expect oil,
good times, freedom to fly—this rat race
we've created—busy ants we destroy
by progress. Slowed down we passed
one birthday, then another in lockdown,
a year science caught up—created
a vaccine—catered to our whims
to serve us back to normal.

Oh Theodore, had you been here
with us these past years—
the crawl-pace filled with emotion,
quiet nights we caught up on reading,
time to write and stay home. That gift—
the world became a still place.
We moved online—opened up vistas—
nuance a keen eye beholds. Is it over,
let me lie down one more time—walk
my neighborhood streets—remember
this new pulse—pause, hear my heart beat—
can we go beyond earning power expulsion—
overdrive stress, everyone mad

with survival of the fittest.
Now is the time for reconsideration
before we wield our way forward,
can we see how we've changed?

Oh Theodore, had you been here
with us these past years—
to question the good COVID has done
for earth—the many lives lost, this purge
nature's retribution to equilibrium,
to regain a stake. We are light beings
who must recognize other ways.
We did our part—stopped
a molecular minute—our pace worn
into submission. Our clock reset.
There is a fine point of precision
to expect death—eyes opened to what is most
valuable—the heart knows—the gut-mind
knows, survival of the fittest not a game
but a life changer. We have buzzed
around like lost bees, tired, seeking
a new hive, and our Queen bee.

Learn To Love

A new world is on its way,
it started at Woodstock, with Vietnam
protests, long hair rebels took off
into the blue sky on motorcycles,
forever nomads, now how many
live in RVs on the move
like Romani travelers, changed
by necessity. Far from the standard
American capitalist lifestyle,
way beyond the reach of the buzz.
We travel through life and time, make a path,
create our heart-home—we carry
each other, hold hands
learn to love.

Waking

late morning (after a long restless
night) blurry eyes focus on the ceiling,
sky in shadows, the clock projects
11:11 neon against the wall

an accusation somewhere vague
in my brain, tainted modern
criminal, off-balance, sleeping-in
11:12 is the turn-key

out of bed into the cool room,
exit the womb between
blanket and sheet, blasted
with air, light and dust
one must cross through
each day with an agenda
(formed, or not) this critical
movement, one world to the next

we traverse our time
fractured, come to terms
but the point is to awaken
alive, to drag our self from
the dead of sleep

Safe Space

There are moments settled
when worry dissipates: in synch,
set, grounded solid on earth, a
sturdy elongated spine rooted
up though my lower back.

Then a shock swings in like
Tarzan on a long tendril, but not
to the rescue, a disrupter–with
bad news–I flinch, cringe,
fold inward, the world tilts.

Then the fall–a deep well
cold damp, clammy skin-crawl,
a wire tightens in my throat,
stability a shadow–I must
slow down, touch earth, find

the smooth stone in my pocket
rub it with my thumb, ask for
what I need–something small.
Today when I spilled into despair,
lost my center, uncertainty flooded,

a part of me knew my cerebral
cortex would come back–my
my toes, fingers, heart and gut
would respond to my plea for calm.
Brain fogged, I start with each

finger–feel the pen, the fabric
against my thigh, my cool cheeks,
a hug across my heart–back doors
into this body, to the safe space
that begins with tactile presence.

The Things I Do Become Calendar

Pure illusion this movement forward, no entourage
or chattel to carry me, what I never said haunts
me with the strongest memories.

No mountains to climb on my current agenda,
the river never crossed was a stone bridge, not a
wooden covered one, how I remembered it.

Trail blaze, to make a new path, geological
maps are helpful, the goal is an illusion.
People talk but what do they say–

impossible to know what anyone means–
sitting with tears your heart brain knows
the answer. Something new must form outside

normal procedure. Yesterday was exactly like
today. It can be difficult to make a new map,
to reconstruct those early years if you did not

keep an outline of your life. Move one day at a
time, let go the mercenary dream, how
much we want but never achieve. Accept

the surprise violets in this long forward
dream. The call of the unspoken, we could have
been closer, or said I love you one more time.

Starting Over

in the running water of time I slipped
over a threshold,   back roads
wide abyss,   deep,   a bird squawks
in the dark night   scattered noise
the pads of my feet   long for ground
this tumble   like combat   to survive
reliance on deep heart   kindness.

I've landed, it seems, a million times
in rooms I grew to love, restructured each life
in a firm grip   despite the fall

unsteady toes flounder to feel land or mud
even sand on a craggy beach,   rocks
in a stream.   A voice calls,   *here*, and reaches
out a warm hand   energy surges through
my body I meld into a new tomorrow.
It worked out. A door opened I could not
have seen. A red bird flickers across the sky.

Do what is possible   reclaim a home   fierce
desire, to be safe   a lock installed, no longer
carrion   for a circling Turkey Vulture.

New York Escape

after Matt Eiford-Schroeder

Everything at once always, said New York City
gloating at how much sits on its solid granite base—
razed so long ago. Its electric lines buried beneath
ground, no ugly wires overhead. We did it all early—
built that subway—one line then the next, we forget
the order of everything once it arrives—here now,
everything in place, in its decay—it was always
perfect at the beginning.

It's hard to leave such an *everything at once always* place
one gets stuck in the wonder, in awe of the clear sky
narrow between skyscrapers, carrier pigeons inbred
for sheer cliffs along an ocean, their DNA recalls—deep
genetics—they taste their insides rotting from old bread
fed to them by an elder on a park bench. One day
they rise free. Some of us escape, resettle, take
a deep breath, mingle with other birds, stand on a true

cliff. No window washers on platforms, no poison
put out to lure an early death. Here there are no white
flour crackers, no easy food that bloats, here we are prey,
we forget that *everything at once always* place,
now with our self, the same life and death, the innate
satisfaction of the familiar. Landed on sheer rock
a cliff over an ocean. We perch.

Letting Go

There are worse things that could happen than disappearing
without a trace, aren't there?
                                                    —Eva Saulitis

I'm letting go of earthly possessions,
      except this book, maybe that book.
After a certain age, there is no need
      for a clunky couch.
Give up the dream of a Queen or a King size
      bed, such inflated desire.
Forgo the new sink fixture, although easy-to-grasp
      handles work better than thick plastic knobs.

Money has its say, there comes a point
      when two hundred dollars is too much to spend.
And you long for a flush bank account, you assert
      life does not require a large footprint.

All life requires is a trace, a roll down the hillside, a sweet
      stalk of wheat to suck, soil beneath your feet.
Earth has its own grief and will buck up against belongings,
      steal them away, only a matter of time.

The trace you leave, that book you wrote
      tomorrow will be left out in the rain, pages curled.
That glass of water you swallowed till half empty,
      you realize the futility of wealth.

How unreal we are against natural forces: fire, rain—
      stars explode—we don't feel their sparks.
The homeless with their pungent bodies dig in the trash,
      cars with shaded windows drive past.

The end is coming fast. No matter how young, now
     is the time to sort out what is necessary.
To make decisions, the yes, the no, to clarify
     the ache we feel for this or that possession.

Those of Us Who Aborted

We came out of broken homes. Our fathers' died or went to jail. There were few role models. We grew used to making our own decisions. Fast early. Distracted into sex. Afraid of sex. Wanting but not wanting. We knew it all. Blown up in our certainty—we would not get caught, until we were. Nothing we could do wrong or right. It wasn't supposed to happen, but it did, and we were lucky to have an escape hatch. Abortion legal so long, fifty years. We had that luxury—took it for granted. We hid our secret—it was shameful what we did—caught, sluts. We might have been raped. We were ruined. We gave it away and it went awry. Determined—no more. We were getting to know our bodies. How the pill made us sick—but kept us safe. The Copper 7 was a trial we could survive. The Dalkon Shield ruined our uterine wall. Some of us survived. Men in our life supported us or left. Our families bent in—or away, deserting us to the streets. Some of us had jobs—others not, we begged and went to work the same day our wombs were scraped. We had a partner with us or a girlfriend or we went alone. We knew women used to die from this and we didn't know if it would kill us—we were babies—some of us had our tonsils removed—ate ice cream. Others never had surgery, didn't know you could walk in and walk out. We were a mess or ultra-confident. We were angry wanting a child but the timing was off. Or we knew this was the right decision. We wanted to believe in something. Mixed with emotions that plagued us—did anybody understand? There was not enough time to make such a decision, but limited time to make it. Weeks. Crunched now, to zero.

II: Unresolved

Until the missing story of ourselves is told,
nothing besides told can suffice:
we shall go on quietly craving it.

–Laura Riding Jackson,
The Telling

1952 Water Dragon

Born in the year airbags were invented,
three of five American families owned
a car. One car. My father drove
twenty miles to work. Dwight Eisenhower
won the election—I didn't know—
nor the Korean war, nor the cold war.
At school in northern Appalachia we didn't do drills,
didn't hide under desks. Sheltered,
we visited family in the city: fun outings,
exhaust fumes smelled sweet.

My family didn't suffer the depression,
grandfather worked, but still:
a child of hoarders,
a child of the nuclear bomb.
Fear in my mother's voice.
Born in a Water Dragon year,
an early boomer, my father wounded,
my uncle a nervous breakdown, in WWII.
My great-great grandfather fought
on the north side of the Civil War.

A patriotic family.
A "Singing in the Rain"
Gene Kelly splash-splash girl-child,
skirting country and city wearing dresses.
Between wars, my father's purple heart
in the attic. He adored me, mother confused me.
Unaware of the many paralyzed by polio.
Dad and I did milk runs to Grandma
after Daddy came home from work.
Mother married at 19, 20 the average in 1952.

How I Came to this World

after Gregory Pardlo

It was leap year, on a Thursday, I was born
     upstate New York, Borsch Belt small town.
To a family of farmers, where covered bridges crossed
     creeks. Twenty miles to the racetrack in
Monticello, our nearest city, where father worked
     for an air conditioning installation firm.
The Evergreens of the Catskills.
     A mother off seeking four-leaf clovers.
Born to arrowheads and quartz, to blueberry
     bushes in back fields. I ran to frogs
and salamanders across stone fences
     through wild woods, no eyes followed me.
It was during the cold war red scare, but I,
     a wild barn child was unaware. Daddy's little girl,
I wore patent leather shoes at Easter and
     blue velvet at Christmas. The cameo necklace
Mother gave me fell into a stream. I was a wild thing
     from go, feeling the velocity of wind. The night
I came a fierce push. I was born clear white,
     pastel perfect skin, with spit-on Irish blood
and German ancestry I was told to never
     acknowledge by a direct line uncle. The year
I came, there was a storm brewing in the guts
     of women to have climaxes they'd never reached.
There was a surge to land on the moon. The
     Atom bomb was introduced from Britain. Born
in the year of the Dragon, I knew it would be rocky,
     not a song in the rain, nor the cotton candy
fun world where mother resided.

Rusty Chain Heritage

The antique cards of my great grandmother,
the photographs of ancestors I did not know,
so much regal furniture, I sat in a closed off
parlor, quiet in a King George chair, looked

across the room at the matching couch,
the grand organ, the gold trimmed tall mirror
with marble at its base, hung full length
between tall windows formally draped.

I loved the quiet in this room, the history I
never understood. The organ no one played,
out of tune, a museum for far away relatives
in England or Holland, mother's side

of the family, who tried to stay wealthy
but exposed to the elements, oxidized
in a slow decline, till it wore thin this familial
chain, clear to inevitable death.

So much no one remembers, two chairs
left, reupholstered, and the mirror, yes, the
mirror, on sister's wall in Philadelphia,
no longer with its marble stand, but it hangs

a view to see ourselves, how we have walked
through to this other side—some of us—who
would be us, long disappeared, those still here
with traces in our blood, on our walls, in the

pictures we grow older and more distant
every decade—this rusty chain still present—
binding like a cross, there is no escape, no matter
the life we live now.

Praying Mantis, in Memory of Louella

My Great Grandmother, Louella,
on my mother's side, lived long
and strong till nearly 98.
In my teens she had a stroke,
lived on our closed-in porch
in Queens. She became my advocate.
What they did was wrong–
forced her to move to the city
from her country farmhouse–
after they found that frozen
praying mantis on her screen door
early spring. An omen they said.

Each summer we drove upstate
to Great Grandma's. Mother and Uncle
grumbled, *she's too old to spend winters alone.*
Then, that praying mantis–
a sign of paralysis–so they moved her
like they moved me–to a concrete
bound world, the city.
She stood up for me, said
it was fine I go on a first date.
She became our neighborhood
window watcher, knew everyone,
every secret on our block.

She told stories, at Kitty Hawk
the first airplane flew like a bird,
stories from the Civil War, how the men
in our family fought, her husband on
the North side, the right side.
We lost so many memories
when we lost Louella.

Ancestor Grounds

In the blue room my ancestors held my fate, their genome
that made me—born to this world soft, gullible, screaming
at the top of my lungs in the face of air—blue veins run
wild, a river coursing its path under a wooden covered
bridge—the dream of good old, what life
                                    was once, never would again.

Here in the blue blood room of my ancestors: a sitting room
with King of England furniture: an organ, royal for a church,
but our heritage in disarray—no one plays the beacon
in the parlor corner. Dark and quiet, curtains drawn, a space
I go to dream, for peace, to sort Great Grandma's antique
                                    cards, stored in a cast iron pot.

I idle hours, safe and quiet, far from the yellow kitchen,
the ongoing upgrades Grandma refuses. Still they install
a refrigerator, indoor plumbing, paint the tin ceiling
half a dozen times in summers that come and go,
make it new—give it a good coat—tin squares embossed,
                                    classic retro redone to a drop down

ceiling, tin belittled. We move fast and far from our regal
bloodline, from Grandmother and her stories. After she passed,
they cleared the kitchen to be a habitat for mice, their skeletons
poured from a smooth walled urn in the back pantry, my scream
loud as the day I arrived, holding the blue inside
                                    demanding my heritage.

Slow Growth

Bombarded by men who could sit hours on
a lake in a boat waiting for a fish to bite.
Patience their virtue—we had few options.

I was a girl in the country who had to save myself,
mother had hands like scissors and a mouth with no words.
Hoping for the best, after we moved, I followed the dream—

rebellion—independence, I escaped into city parks,
crushed pennies on railroad tracks. Nothing was right.
I said no to unwanted advances, forging a path.

My dreams grew and the clouds cleared—I had to get small
before I could get big—dreams squelched too easy after Father
died, but there is something about moving on despite

all odds against. Miracles live on the horizon—a tiny seed
I could have discarded, but I held it in my dark center, it had to
germinate a long time, it was cheerless and mournful for years.

With no other option but to press forward, it finally bloomed
like an orchid that took forever, then stunned me with love.

Loosely Knit

We have ancestors we can no
longer name, faded photographs
their identities buried with great
grandmothers, aunts and uncles
who took their memories with

them, each death we lost history–
our family line unraveled–I had
to let go, move across the country.
My sister brought us new blood,
a son, adopted from Vietnam–

he brought rich silk tapestries
of rice fields and holds our family
name–a fresh embroidery to rethread
our fabric once rich with story. A ghost
aunt, I live three thousand miles away,

visit every two years, words on a
holiday card, a gift each birthday,
such distant commodities offered.
I do not know who he is edging into–
it is not right to criticize a sister's

mothering, or to question his
upbringing–we remain a small dying-
out family. I hang unwoven, a loose
thread, keeper of blurry photographs
my nephew will never phantom.

The Night of the Stroke

Visiting my sister in Philly to meet
my new nephew, adopted from Vietnam,
my sister and I eat spaghetti with meat sauce,
Mom and her new grandson rest upstairs–
a crash and a thud crackle through the baby monitor–
we find Mom on the floor–she waves her hand,
shakes her head, *no*, but we call 911.
I sit next to her on the bathroom floor, hold her hand,
my sister sits to calm her new son. Emergency
Medics come fast, strap her to a mat. I whisper,
She has schizophrenia. A fact my sister won't tell,
but she rides alongside Mom in the ambulance.
I finish my spaghetti, get a ride to the hospital
with a neighbor. In ICU a CT scan shows damage,
she can't talk, there is concern about clots
in her neck breaking loose, we notice a catheter
up her urethra–her heart beeps across a monitor,
our eyes watch the beat, a nurse asks about insurance,
mentions complications. Says, *Medicare won't cover
complex care*. Adamant, I demand a social worker.

Boys Prefer Trucks

My sister brought home a boy, she agreed
to whichever sex came first. Her surprise,
boys really do like trucks, like girls like dolls,
it's not a myth she insists, *I did nothing*

to encourage this love of every truck he sees.
He bounces in the car, points his finger at
garbage trucks, tractor trailer trucks, cargo
trains, she emphasizes, *boys love trucks and*

trains. She insists she had no influence, but
she bought him a hand carved wooden train set
in Pike Place Market, spent more than I make
in a day. He's a boy-king traveling the world

with my sister, the lawyer, growing him up
international: Paris, Vienna, Italy, and when he turned
nine they visited his home country, Vietnam, to see if
he had interest in connecting, he did not. He's

Americanized with a fleet of toy rigs, he plays
basketball. His aunt, we have nothing in common.
A geek on his computer, his phone, he builds robots.
Off to college, he's ready to truck around the world.

Family of Random Churches

Mother did not find me holy,
>*Holy! Holy! Holy!*
>Allen Ginsberg wrote.

He proclaimed our world holy—
to the asshole—a word
I never heard my mother use
till I rebelled—and she cursed me
with words I never knew she knew.

A church goer, she sought
peace of mind at a Baptist church—
>dunked, she insisted
>I get dunked, too,

her way to save me—my head
immersed, my hair ruined. No,
I said—enough—I was sprinkled
as a baby, at my father's

Methodist church.
>Firm against her intrusion—
>I found my own church,

Congregationalist. I was never an easy
child, she said. Nothing smooth
between us. After Dad died
she gave up. Moved us
to her childhood home in the city,

let go her independence—
her driver's license, swimming.
Unable to live alone—the same way
I need a partner. Avoidant, I resist
>love, push away anyone
>I need. Mother and I

never compatible, each buried
under pain–

we lost the love of our lives.
Paralyzed from a stroke
at a nursing home,
she settled into watching Fox
        became Fundamentalist.
        Our Holy war over.

Unresolved Mother

When there was never a mother to turn to
but you needed a mother. When you had to become
your own mother, answer your own questions,

learn to survive without a functional guide.
Each day held hope, something would change.
She might snap out of the world she lived in

join you, have a mother-to-daughter conversation.
She might change her clothes, put on a clean dress,
wash the butter out of her hair, that she uses

to protect against hair stylists. Maybe the mother
you dreamed would emerge. Now orphaned,
you regret you weren't kind enough, you wish

you'd known earlier about schizophrenia, internal
voices, and why she would not bathe. Wish you'd
insisted she drink water that hot day of her stroke.

After Mother's Death

My mother never enters at the right
time, even in my dreams.
It's been that way since I've known her.

She was asleep on my arrival
and had nothing to say for years
I had to love her–there are rules

that sit in the gut, how we love,
regurgitate, turn sour,
bile pushes against the flap

keeping it in place–
that love
a dandy mess of our insides–

we can't escape even when we've
grown old, you see when she died
there was a long

complicated grief and panic rising,
there was no control in this body
that pushed hard against her a lifetime.

The Moment of Diagnosis

after Lucia Perillo

For now, I'll just stand in the courtyard.
For news is news   and I have the wisdom of the *Zero Step.*
The *do nothing step*,   the stillness to listen inside,   the now
to gather and hold this body erect,   to stay quiet and wait,
drink water,   watch the sky and the trees grounded in the
earth,   to know what to hold onto.

Sure,   anger comes and fear,   but
these trees guide a hidden disease.

There was a moment I did not know, different yet the same–
                    For now, I'll just stand in the courtyard.

The diagnosis hit like a tailgate strike,   a scathing jolt,
a wake-up crash,   whiplash,   but there is a way
to forgive–to stand with trees–to grow a gradual
acceptance,   a sliver matures in stillness,   time passes
moves on to what transpires next,   on a tree leaves come and go,
this process   cycling to a calling   that opened to a career
that came and went,   I survive like the trees,   in their daily standing.

It makes sense,   this emotional stew that stormed my life–
a personal study–how to midwife the specter of death.

Grateful to the trees that absorb pain, they would accept even
my blood if I had to bleed. I stand today   one of the lucky ones.
Me and the trees,   the trees and I
in the wind,   in this courtyard.

The Soft Middle Space During a Pandemic

To go insane
I would talk to my mother
daily–and she's dead
so this makes it easier.

If I had not taken the woman's
hand to help her down from the ledge
where she sat when she
asked for help, I would be bereft,

there was no one for miles
that warm morning and yes
there were already Corona
virus warnings: don't touch,

wash your hands, stay inside.
But I reached out, took her swollen
red hand, soft and warm to touch.
She thanked me after she moved

to the sidewalk with my
support, grateful, *thank you*
in a low vulnerable whisper
no virus separated us.

I would be delusional
if I believed myself invulnerable
or impenetrable to disease
or to this virus, if too calm

while the world panics–
it's hard to stay centered, easier
to be preoccupied but not ignore,
to stay in that soft middle space.

It was a frenetic party at the piano bar
the young women celebrating,
sparkling at their table: dayglo pink,
neon blue, jet black, shock yellow,

and manic orange hair, drinking
martinis and dancing to the music,
they were not sheltered-in-place
and we were travelers celebrating

with locals on the Riverwalk
enjoying these moments before
the seriousness of separation began.
It is absurd to enter a quarantine

too easy, to not expect to get sick
to assume you will not die
while hundreds of thousands are infected
and notices of death increase

on your Facebook feed.
I came back to my hotel
and washed my hands after
helping the woman step down

from the ledge, my fear did not
stop me, she might have sat there
forever and that is inhumane,
for now, weeks later no one touches.

I talk to my dead mother
tell her I'm okay, that the streets
are empty, somehow she knows
this is strange, she understands

my fascination with the streets,
how I never stayed home, but
ran away, far away from her
searching for safety, for other.

Social Distance

We need each other every single
day, month, year, generation.
Interdependent, we reach out,
barn raise with our neighbors.
Community, we lift each other up,
gather round a fire, a hearth, sing,
organize a union, speak unfettered
our worry and love.

We travel across boundaries, move ageless
like cowboy poets spreading news region-
to-region. The call for knowledge
lifted from truth and source, a wide web–
little insistence on independence–
we understand how frail each human. The idea
of a superhero manifests in good deeds,
Lassie barked, *Help, he needs help,*
and there was a rescue.

How can I learn to lean on others
when touch is extracted from my bones?
When I no longer care who sees me at my
worst. What deep seated fear rolls me
from a plethora of necessary help from another?
My partner rubs my back with healing herbs,
he, the only one I expect support from–the one
who is there, trusted. We have a couple bubble,
faith and love, but how many have even one

person in these hazardous times?
My friend with asthma, suffocated by smoke,
left, took a plane to Chicago, then a plane
to Portland, Maine, with no plan. With
little money, no credit card, no one to meet her

at either airport. She used the last of her cash
for this grand escape so she could breathe,
fires encroaching her home.

She asked for donations I wish I had to give.
This is a time of risk and daring for those
on the edge of survival. Our world on the slope
of decline, we roll into mire, claw through mud
to the top of a hill already crowded, those
who slip and die the earth accepts as filler.

Cento For My Younger Sister with Multiple Myeloma

There have been monsters under my heart since I was born.
You see, I had no sister when I was little
a dove that nests in Paris's walls
has warmed a cuckoo's egg–

I am in her like dust in a tornado,
night in a star, ice in a glacier.
I love my sister I need my sister
to wade in the dark night water,

to sneak in and out of back doors
saying the spell under my breath
that no life is slight enough to pass
how "Fuck you" becomes a love song.

I predict that losing you, specifically,
will be too much to bear. You are a species
                    that knows it will go extinct.
This is how I will let go of loss,
by carrying you with me.

After a hug, the between is holdable,
fortune-tell a sense of longing and loss.
I cannot love without a sister
I whisper, *How long do we have?* to no one in particular.

A Lifetime Missing My Sister

—Sarah Kay, *In the House with No Doors*

We'd always been tight against
each other, a sliver of air
between us, the world swirling—
together in the center, safe
holding tight, a mirror to look
inside. Sister, where did you go?

Which doorway did you exit,
I left first, the oldest, forced to escape—
the sheer velocity of those winds
we buoyed against in the family home—
our belly buttons torn separate, cut
like leaving mother—a cold scissors—

brutal metal on soft flesh—
I mourned for you when Mom
threatened to send you away—
I left you behind to stand on your own
without me—would you survive?
What tools in that mire to continue?

The long years till you stood
on your own feet—off to college—
how proud that you graduated,
our beat in tune taking steps
in this world—sisters—separated
by a family splintered against us.

Not even a doorknob between us
yet we opened that door, found
a way out. Bound together by blood

the long missing we suffered, COVID
years, your bones disintegrating.
Life moves steady onward without

each other. My closeness to you
way too close for your comfort,
three thousand miles distant, our
doorknob a steady connection,
we grew in the same womb—a knot
of love, a distant ring we hear.

III: Revolutionary

*Hope is perhaps simply a stance toward the world,
finally, a stance of participation, or inseparability.*

—Mark Doty,
Heaven's Coast

Lost Wanna Die Moments

It's a long road living with AIDS,
a constant surprise why I continue
when so many died. My body strong,
not exhausted. I lived on the right

side of town, not like my friend next
to a migrant worker building, drunken
brawls, bodies thrown out windows,
bloody wounds late at night.

I sat alone vomit spewing, pressured
skull ache, over-the-toilet puking–
years I took that cyclic birth control
pill, each month a sour hell.

I prayed, not because I believed,
but a call of agony, take me please.
Then continued till the next wanna
die–that spiral with wretched

days, mood fluctuations, sleep
a wax, a wane, a wind-swept dame.
Shingles, like a lightning bolt–
nervous system fried–rapid

rupture, pierced eye made me cry
please let me die. My body defied
calls for ease. Like Sisyphus
I trudged up mountains, ready

to fall down. Did you hear me god?
Your directions weren't clear,
you said take the dirt road, watch
for the barn–used to be a barn

felled in a fire in 89—disappeared
like the too many gone. We live
in a vanishing world: loves of our
life, languages, species, ice floes.

My favorite Kosher Deli—COVID
closed—piled pastrami sandwiches
with Russian dressing, gone. My
cries to die circle like clock hands,

the waning moon, a steady tick tock
metronome. Yet I stand, a miracle,
on the road to the next mountain,
despite my near burnt down barn.

Northwest Mineral Springs

Seeking renowned remote hot
springs, wild space to soak naked—
we found one near the Columbia
River—back woods, known to locals,
warned of the gnarly path, reminded
to pay the parking fee. Heated pools
of mineral water we sat with a traveler
who lived at The Farm in Tennessee.
A rare summer day of freedom—
glints of silver in the waterfalls
across from our sequestered rock hovel—
salmon jumping upstream—
interloper from the east coast, could I
believe my eyes? We moved closer to see
their silver shimmers. Oblivious to us
they swam instinctual and urgent
in cold icy water to spawn and die.
We dipped our toes into their running
river, satisfied, we returned to our soak—
a mere mile from Carson Hot Springs
where they piped this very water
into white porcelain tubs and charged
a fee for what we indulged for free.

Bad Mouth Tang

Anywhere I go–
starting a new job,
walking into a workshop ready to learn a new lexicon,
traveling in a foreign country,
or waking fresh on a foggy morning,
convinced I've left my old baggage behind.

No one wants the suitcase I carry
filled with what feels important–
photos, memories, losses,
a moonlit eve I smoked my first joint,
a neighbor who used me
and I used him.

Dozens of sex stories,
a bunch of female-living-in-a-man's-world shit
even I cannot stand.
Yeah, I've left it behind
shoved it under the bed and hope no one finds it.
It will free itself in a curse one day–

only I and a few I once knew
have seen how I rock a bad mouth motherfucker–
my Queens tang will give me away
at some high class party–
I've never belonged, my stockings always had a run,
my toes hurt, my gangly legs didn't know where to land,

so I stood stock still.
Always a fresh start,
unexperienced, ready to learn
to grasp and figure it out–
who are the right people to ask–
to smile, to survive.

To Take a Life

She wanted to know how metal
intersected with skin blood bones.

Fascinated with car accidents
the abrasive crunch, airbags

concave chest, air exhaled, and
how we die. She watched a cat

expire after her car slammed into
him. Heartbeat on her tongue—no

answer—what to do with a body.
A voice screaming inside

some little girl's cat she murdered—
tears in his white fur, body turning

cold and rigid in her arms, pee
and shit a cascade onto her fine

wool jacket, more answers
than she ever deserved.

Radical Places

There used to be days free from AIDS
they were irresponsible days, free as the gay
men finding themselves in the late 70s,
gay bars a thing, the lesbian bars full.

Were we internally homophobic—
                            because of this culture?
It was a mind-explosion time
I remember that first thrill
meeting a real lesbian,
going to my first
lesbian bar, enlightening nights

the thrill of dress up and party,
the irresponsibility to have fun,
but we paid bills, went to
consciousness raising groups,
found our people
our writers: Adrienne Rich, Audre Lorde,

we fought repression, burned our bras
in these days of freedom
before the gay cancer,
before my bisexuality returned,
before the change to assimilation,
but I knew I could never be straight again,
even if I appeared so,
would never marry, would never
have the children I didn't want,
                                            I knew
and it didn't feel irresponsible, it felt
                                            right
to be in this radical place, it felt new and exciting
to consider marrying a gay man for his green

card, a choice to make and I, responsible Virgo,
decided No, I did not want legal entanglement
even if I wanted my gay friend to have the right
to live here, certain things we have to say no to,
like saying yes
        it comes from deep inside.

I've Lived Through One War

I've had my share of the *I'm dying* lament
I'll not go there with this new pandemic
I lived through one war, AIDS. Worked
and lived through death up-close—

people take risks—bug-chasers fucked
to get HIV—that old story. Citizens
throw Corona parties to get sick, build
immunity, they make decisions irrespective

of rules or science—meet with a friend,
walk in a park—conscientious, I will
shelter in place within reason, unafraid.
My body strong despite a retrovirus

I've learned to live with thirty years.
No known reason why I survived. People
criticize those who exercise free will, speak
with judgement from fear, become vigilante

citizens, fight with store clerks who request
they wear a mask. In the Philippines they shoot
offenders of shelter in place. We must ask
new questions, find unconventional answers,

remember our history, listen to those who
survived stigma and shame. It's time
for massive change before we proceed.
Our planet, slow now with clear skies.

What They Mean When They Say Worried Well

When I learned my status, therapy
seemed a good plan. One appointment
and I knew he was not the right fit,
he told me I would have to stay where
I worked. What? And then he said
I was one of the *worried well*. What?

This didn't fit my vision, it felt
presumptive, a lie, and what the fuck
was *worried well*? I looked it up.
Now with COVID-19 I hear
this phrase again on the news
for those not sick but anxious.

This broad stroke category wipes
away feelings, it tidies and organizes,
You're fine, one of the *worried well*.
In fact, you might make trouble, take
too many tests, use supplies others
need. Back then HIV meant death,

the phrase confused me, was I well?
Hard to know with a retrovirus inhabiting
my body. Everyone lives on a spectrum
of health and neuroticism. Worried well,
two contradictory words, an erasure that
negates, gives you back the problem—

your worry—if you weren't so worried
you'd be fine. Well, I'm fine, less anxious
about this new virus than most around me—
I survived a deadly disease thirty plus years—
became a therapist, and will not label those
who shake with fear. Death is a well

we fall into, and worry is a prophylaxis
like a placebo–to help us grow strong,
take precautions, find answers. I found my way
in the maze–friends and chosen family died.
My web broke with each new death. We must sit
and listen, hold gentle our brothers and sisters

ask what they need, how they plan to
to get where they're going, despite illness
and fear. Find channels that soothe. Breath.
Words. Writing through the nervous system
onto the page. Send anxiety into the earth.
Move on the continuum–sickness to

wellness–find the mindful present, feel
the body in toes and feet, seek calm.
I never returned to that therapist. It was 1990,
I got a Masters, moved to my next job,
and the next, opened a private practice.
My retrovirus and I are well, not worried.

At a Time Like This

new options explode, we download
Zoom, everything moves online,
We review the rules and protocol.

Swamped as usual, my building
being resided by construction
workers, who are essential.

I write a poem a day for National
Poetry Month, feel a surge of
possibility for change, worry

about the election, concern for the
homeless, how others will survive.
Water turned off in city fountains,

no public bathrooms open,
parks closed, except they are full–
we are a mess, but life continues,

food in my fridge. I add herbs
to strengthen my host immune system,
so when I get this virus, I will survive.

My herbal mentor said, we will get COVID-19,
we must build our body strong.
Grateful for this life we must fight back

the way the community fought
during AIDS. We must learn from them
in this new age. We need ways to win,

like they did in the 80s and 90s.
We cannot lose our advances.
My heart hurts for those who live alone.

COVID Years of Lost Family Time

My sister's diagnosis, Multiple Myeloma:
radiation, chemo, a stem cell transplant,
hip surgery. I sent healing, ceded my usual
visit these closed down years.

My partner's mother in decline—
jaundiced at 92—a tube scraped throat—
she said, *no more*—stopped eating,
refused tests. Twenty-four hours

he and his brothers sat at her bedside
with home hospice. December a swell
with her exit. An ice storm barred an easy
trip home. Family loomed large in distant

cities: protection, safety prominent.
We held energy through time. Grateful
to those close who did what we could not.
The trial of illness on top of illness, our job

to stay strong, vaccinate. He had no choice
but to go—I, no choice but to stay—we carried
responsibility to survive. My sister I will see
in an unknown future, under a semblance

of normal, make my way east, aim for
my nephew's graduation. Her travel
bug returning, without a wheelchair, she
adjusts to a cane. Her lifetime extended,

our future limited. My mother-in-law's time
expired, she missed a final family visit.
Her older sister died at home after the news,
said, *I can leave now.* More family gone

these years then in our forty together.
Planes overloaded, his luggage lost,
he drove a long night north to return
home Christmas morning.

What Gives Hope

The miracle might be we emerge from this
a better world with a clearer vision, higher
priorities, a closer connection to each other;

that we might learn to live together in peace,
a new emphasis on healing the pain
our ancestors perpetuated with slavery.

We've been isolated in this pandemic, thrown
online to meet. Contact our most important
social soothing, cyber space not the body-

to-body we yearn, nuance obscured with distance.
Awash in protest against condoned police violence,
still, some are hopeful. It is clear now, essential

workers are not expendable. We return
our blood to the earth by rule of militaristic volition,
let us be drained like slaughtered deer. Or,

die in hospitals from COVID-19, intubated.
In the streets, we have always died. Our blood,
our breath, obstructed with no mercy, a clamp

on the poor with no clout—unlike those who
prosper from crisis. We, the little ones with jobs lost,
income gone, family dead from systemic violence,

these pressured times we've always lived through.
Yet some have hope and fire to burn, the young
who knew Obama their first eight years.

Following in his legacy, yet-to-lead on the front line
of change that is coming. And oh, to have
their fresh votes, their wisdom, their vision.

Rules on Life from a Green Witch

I.

1. Find someone to instruct.
2. Prevention. Prevention. Prevention:
    2.a. Oat grass infusion;
    2.b. Springtime nettles, cooked like spinach;
    2.c. Lick the dew of dawn.
Appendix: Spoonful's of organic earth while crawling through childhood.
3. Fermentation; like a God.
4. Remember, ancestors in the old country never visited doctors.
5. Write one sentence per day: ordain it a poem.
6. Yell when you feel like it, smile when you don't; scream to release.
7. Expect surprises.
8. You are water, let your body have its own movement.
9. Your umbilical cord shifts earth mother to universe: rebirth is a biological need.
10. Breathe through your nose: in, out, in, out, calm slow; feel; will breath into each toe.
11. Your beliefs make who you become. A friend nurtures who you will become.
12. Silence is sacred.
13. A coven number for a perfect circle.
14. Accept what you want, even if you are not ready.
Disclaimer: most everything is your life depends on where you are born, to whom and into what class or clan.

II.

She takes slow steps toward the street.
You wait and give her your hand.
She says, *Life is hard, so you have to love.*
Wise, she says it again

holding tight to your arm.
You walk her across the street, say, *Thank you.*

III.

Don't wait till anyone dies to be your true self.

A Witch, Despite

How does a woman escape the payback
from a male-bent society?

Our tribe, with its winding history
of persecution, so many of us
burned at the stake.

Implicit in the word witch: female,
a broom, a caldron brew of herbs, secret
formulas that heal–from land we owned,
once the commons.

How dare we live independent!
The men, their crux a cross of disciplinary
action–to punish such brazen hussies,
remove us from their sacred earth.

Insistent in our right to property,
men kill like the bandits they consider brave,
retaliation a force to burn any Joan of Arc.
Thousands of us lost to their fires.

Brutal, this world enforced by men–
who stole our land–thieves with no mercy.
Still, we strive beyond their control–such power
with their cache of ships and tea,

we hold close each remedy–sit quiet
with a pregnant woman–it's the sitting with
we do best, slow down to witness and heal,
a hug, a mug of tea, an infusion, a soup, handed

oh-so-careful, to another in need. This wealth,
our silent way a path so different it spurns hatred–
we understand wisdom emanates
from the smallest, simplest seed.

Through the Lens: 7 Revolutionary Practices

She looks at the world with her mean stare.

> He and I meet for tea. On the wall is a framed photo,
> the cover of a book: *Anxious to Please: 7 Revolutionary*
> *Practices for the Chronically Nice*
> So many people I know need to double confirm,
> but not this friend.

She has eyes that penetrate with distrust.

> We sit in the tea house.
> *One must show up.*
> I order herbal Chai, he orders Snow White, a green tea.

She rarely wants anything to do with anyone.

> What bugs me as we sit and drink our tea
> is his dust-laden eyeglasses.
> *One must be present when one shows up.*
> I sit wondering how he can see clearly,
> this gravely distracts me.

She guards her words, a dragon in front of her castle-home.

> We talk, but I don't mention the dust.
> *One must keep the commitment one makes.*
> He and I are friends, yet never before met for tea.

She's wary of people; has names for them: grabbers,
swindlers, child thieves.

> Secretly, I think this book on the chronically nice
> must be meant for me.
> *One must keep one's word.*

The question, how can he see clearly,
is blatantly consuming me.

She'll bark and bite and scratch your eyes out like a cat, a lion.

I find it hard to relax into the now with my Zen cup of tea.
Be here now.
He said he'd be here and he is. But am I?

She's used to the fight, you can see it in her untamed hair.

How nice do I have to be? Certainly, I'm distracted
from the moment.
One must say what one has to say.
Another question puzzles me,
how well do I really know this friend?

She's used to sitting on curbs alongside the sidewalk.

I clean my eyeglasses obsessively each and every day.
Lost wondering about the habits people cultivate.
How can he see clearly with dusty lenses?

She's grown up fast and fighting.

Can I rely on someone with dust-laden glasses?
Breathe.
A micro fiber cloth in my bag, I watch his eyes
through the dust.

She won't allow herself to be pushed around.

I wonder about the *7 Revolutionary Practices.*
I take my glasses off to see even clearer,
pour yet another cup of tea.

New Age Wonder

Make a ritual.
Gems heal—find a petrified tree,
a quartz crystal in a creek—
reminders of wonder and belief.

Life force spirals—
find solace in water,
in stone, in gentle rainfall,
breathe petrichor released from earth.

Touch a moss laden nurse log.
Feel the pulse of the moon,
the rising of the sun,
star glitter in the sky—
elemental, essential—
a world your body understands.

Hair Ritual

Gather your hair into a soft handkerchief,
shape it into a nest, take it to the
wild earth on a full moon and plant it.

Watch to see what grows, what strange
life may spring from dead cell strands.
There is nothing more valuable than

recreation of life, do this ritual each month.
Ask the universe forgiveness till there is no
hair on your head, no garden in your yard.

Wise Women Herbal Tradition Self-Care Quest

a sonnet tiara

i.

Blind-sided, I stop to hold myself still.
Despite the dark I trust and dance
in unknown waters with slowed-down
movement, arms stretched, a leggings-day,
comfort in a field seeking what soothes
this frayed nervous system. Start with a
ceramic cup to wrap my hands around—
chai, to boost clarity and insight, stop
absorb the heat, acknowledge this time
is the only time despite the stress-hum,
the high-strung eruptions in the world.
I feel my toes, walk onward and listen.
Tree ghosts answer my invisible
questions that float in dark hollows.

ii.

Questions that float in dark hollows–
recessed knowledge of herbs in my cells,
what works well within this body.
Brushing against oats, I hear a whisper,
an ancient wise call from work-horses
whose steady nerves pulled their weight,
consistent strength from what they ate.
There is a wise woman inside. She
understands the nutrition of ritual,
what the plants provide, how they give back
what they take from this earth, how minerals
infuse health through preparation,
prevent illness long before it starts. She's on
a pilgrimage to heal without regret.

iii.

A pilgrimage to heal without regret,

I flutter forward, rustling leaves

offer answers on this golden path.

I taste and harvest bountiful weeds

from nature's wild space, I glow

in sunlight. Give thanks to each cutting,

leave the mother–the tallest ancestor–

say a prayer, bestow my gratitude.

This is time away from busy, time-in

to find myself and my ally plants

to sustain this life into the future.

This quiet where fairies dance and sing

secrets revealed: willow is strongest

during a storm, a twig of willow falls.

iv.

During a storm, a twig of willow falls.

Chewing it, my headache disappears,

ancient ritual of my grandmother

passed on in stories from childhood.

How do I know? Time is universal.

We carry our history in our bones

and mouth, that oral cavity canal—

throat to sphincter—secrets of the body

formulated into science. Foxglove

killed a man, speeded up his heart

now we have Digitalis. Careful,

do not confuse foxglove with comfrey,

that bone knit plant that weaves together

any broken bone from its poultice.

V.

Any broken bone from its poultice,

comfrey will heal like a dream—

miracle plant that scares people.

Wise women have never been afraid,

their anecdotal evidence is strong.

Lost in skepticism, it's hard facing

those with so much authority, backed up

with research from what they stole.

Sensitive in the fray of rules

and regulations, many knocked down,

frightening reality in a world

where people suffer too long, despite

the allies they could use to heal.

Blind-sided, I stop to hold myself still.

Vashon Writing Residency

From my window I watch Canadian
geese on the lawn alongside Quartermaster
Harbor. The couple walks daily, pecking
grass, seeking food, holding each other
company, till one day they have an argument–
squawking, the wings on one flails wide
haranguing their spouse. What is wrong
between them to set their universe askew?
Easter Sunday rain pours down. In my room,
I transcended the deluge, diligent working on
edits. Waves choppy on the harbor, a five
mile inlet filled with pollution years ago
from a plant in Tacoma–the push of the sea
knocks against the floating dock. In this shallow
harbor no marine traffic passes. Signs warn
not to harvest toxic shellfish. Ducks, Canadian
geese, and osprey can't read–so they feast,
broken shells litter the spit.

I let go my goal to harvest Dandelion
when I learn the soil in paradise is toxic,
only raised beds are used to grow food.
I enjoy the beauty–the daily sky,
each sunset, the rise and fall of the shoreline,
safe in a well-built house. We four share
a solid commitment to our art, indulged
in luxury, far from busy cluttered lives.
We nap when needed, welcome
the nurturance we give each other–
shared dinners–feasts of conversation–
growing a closer bond to our work.

There was a time

we stood together
close, with our laughter
and serious expressions–
a long hug for solace.

We were one as a group–
memories we hold:
sitting over tea, picnics,
fairs, potlucks, garage sales.

We laughed till we cried.
We made love for hours.

Found each other at art festivals,
open houses, plays, music venues,
and concerts. We beat drums
at rallies, formed parades,
danced disco till the bar closed.

We need a new world, it is time
to make change, for the next
generations to take over.

So many good dying–
but there is no end to good.

We went to workshops in person
did yoga, contact dancing,
bought gym memberships, traveled,
gathered round a fire, sat at a Seder.

We sang and prayed together.

Now, slowed down,
we move toward each other again.

Notes

"The Moment of Diagnosis": The Zero Step is the first of the Wise Woman Tradition Steps of Healing.

"Cento For My Younger Sister with Multiple Myeloma": This cento is composed of lines from Devon Miller-Duggan, Jennifer D. Brock, Samantha Pious, Kristina Morgan, Sadie Dupuis, Courtney Lund O'Neil, Aaron Wander, Bethany Reid, Aracelis Girmay, Sarah Vapp, Christina MR Norcross, Sarah Dickenson Snyder, Kai Coggin, Rilke (translator Bly), and Joan Kwon Glass.

Acknowledgements & Gratitude

Thank you to following literary journal and anthologies for publishing poems from this collection, sometimes in earlier versions:

Anti-Heroin Chic: "Safe Space," "Rules on Life from a Green Witch," "Letting Go," "Slow Growth," "Bad Mouth Tang," "After Mother's Death," "Lost Wanna Die Moments"

Drip Lit Mag: "Family of Random Churches"

Ethel: "Radical Places"

Feels Blind Literature: "Unresolved Mother," nominated for a Pushcart Prize

Ghost City Press: "New York Escape"

Hags on Fire: "Letting Go"

Humanism Evolving through Arts and Literature: HEAL: "Cento for My Younger Sister with Multiple Myeloma"

I, Enheduanna: "There was a time"

Journal of the Plague Year: "I've Lived Through One War," "What They Mean When They Say Worried Well," "Daily Caution During a Pandemic"

Mad Swirl: "The Things I do Become Calendar"

Mooky Chick: "Starting Over," "Wise Woman Herbal Tradition Self-Care Quest"

Oddball Magazine: "Pupal Soup"

The Poeming Pigeon: "Loosely Knit"

Poetry and COVID: "That Soft Middle Space During a Pandemic"

Red Elk Review: "Praying Mantis, in Memory of Louella"

Seattle Review of Books: "Waking," Rusty Chain Heritage," "How I Came to this World"

The Seattle Star: "Through the Lens: 7 Revolutionary Practices"

Verse Versal: "The Night of the Stroke," "Boys Prefer Trucks"

Voices in the Wind: "To Take a Life"

Wellspring Literary Journal: "The Moment of Diagnosis"

Writing in a Woman's Voice: "Ancestor Grounds"

Anthologies
COVID, *Isolation and Hope: Artists Respond to the Pandemic*, edited by Rafael Alvarado, Consuelo G. Flores and Richard Modiano, Finishing Line Press, 2021: "At a Time Like This," "What Gives Hope"

A Guide to Creative Writing and the Imagination, Kris Saknussemm, Routledge, 2022: "Bus Stop in San Antonio: AWP Off Site"

Poets Speaking to Poets: Echoes and Tributes, edited by Nicholas Fargnoli and Robert Hamblin, Ars Omnia Press, 2021: "How I Came to this World"

The Queer Movement Anthology of Literature, edited by B.B.P. Hosmillo, Sarah Clark, and Mark Anthony Cayanan (press forthcoming): "The Moment of Diagnosis"

Residencies & Writing Programs
Thank you to Mineral School, Vashon Island Residency, and Jack Straw Writers' Program for time and support.

Gratitude
A huge thank you Lana Hechtman Ayers. In the early 2000s she gave me the seed of belief that my poems would be published in book form. I'm grateful for her support and that she chose my manuscript for a MoonPath Press publication. It is a great honor to have a book from this prestigious press that Lana built. And thank you to Tonya Namura for her beautiful design.

Thank you to Marcia Meier who started an online writing group at the beginning of COVID, aptly named Writing Through the Apocalypse. Many of the poems in this book originated in this friendly and supportive group of writers.

With special gratitude to poets and artists John Burgess, Deborah Woodard, Priscilla Long, Ann Tweedy, and Clare Johnson. I'm grateful to the many wonderful poets and artists who never give up.

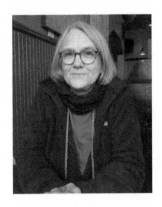

About the Author

Julene Tripp Weaver, a psychotherapist and writer in Seattle, has three prior poetry collections; *truth be bold–Serenading Life & Death in the Age of AIDS* (Finishing Line Press, 2017), which won the Bisexual Book Award, four Human Relations Indie Book Awards, and was a finalist for the Lambda Literary Awards; *No Father Can Save Her*, (Plain View Press, 2011); and a chapbook, *Case Walking: An AIDS Case Manager Wails Her Blues*, (Finishing Line Press, 2007).

Her poems have appeared in many journals including: *HEAL, Autumn Sky Poetry, Oye Drum, Poetry Super Highway, As it Ought To Be,* and elsewhere. Recent anthologies include: *Rumors Secrets & Lies: Poems about Pregnancy, Abortion & Choice, I Sing the Salmon Home, Writing Through the Apocalypse, The Power of the Feminine I: poems from the feminine perspective, Volume 2,* and *Nerve Cowboy Selected Works 2004-2012.*

Her third poetry book, *truth be bold*, empowered her to start writing a memoir about her life and work as a long term survivor. She is an 'Artivist' in the Through Positive Eyes Project sponsored by The Gates Discovery Center and UCLA Art and Global Health. The goal is to eliminate stigma about AIDS by sharing stories. She was a Jack Straw Writing Fellow (2023). Essay publications include: *The Guardian, Hags on Fire, The Muse (McMaster University), Mollyhouse,* which nominated her essay for a Pushcart. Her essay, "Babes With AIDS," about being one of the founders of the Babes Network, a peer support organization for women living with HIV, won Honorary Mention for the Christopher Hewitt Award in Nonfiction, *A&U (AIDS & Understanding) Magazine.*

She has received support from Centrum, the University of Washington's Helen Riaboff Whiteley Center, Mineral School, Vashon Artists in Residence, and Hypatia-in-the-Woods.

Website: julenetrippweaver.com; Instagram: @julenet.weaver

Printed in the USA
CPSIA information can be obtained
at www.ICGtesting.com
LVHW090826220624
783638LV00006B/641